Budget Dinner Cookbook

2ⁿᵈ Edition

35 Affordable Recipes to Feed Your Family Any Night of the Week!

by Olivia Rogers

Copyright © 2017 By Olivia Rogers
All rights reserved. No part of this book may be reproduced in any form without permission in writing from the author. No part of this publication may be reproduced or transmitted in any form or by any means, mechanic, electronic, photocopying, recording, by any storage or retrieval system, or transmitted by email without the permission in writing from the author and publisher.
For information regarding permissions write to author at Olivia@TheMenuAtHome.com
Reviewers may quote brief passages in review.

Please note that credit for the images used in this book go to the respective owners. You can view this at:
TheMenuAtHome.com/image-list

Olivia Rogers
TheMenuAtHome.com

Table of Contents

Introduction 5

1. Green Beans in Coconut Milk 6

2. Minestrone Soup with Macaroni 8

3. Chili Beans with Pasta 10

4. Tuna Spaghetti with Tomatoes and Garlic 12

5. Beef and Vegetable Stew 14

6. Garlic-Herb Beef Roast 17

7. Paella in a Flash 19

8. Baked Mushroom-Chicken Curry Rice 21

9. Red Rice Soup with Beef 24

10. Stir-Fried Shrimp Hofan 26

11. Corned Beef Hearty Soup 28

12. Meatloaf Pasta Parmigiana 30

13. Luncheon Meat Katsudon 33

14. Seafood Fried Rice 36

15. Cajun Pork Chops with Gravy 38

16. Chicken Barbecue with Java Rice 40

17. Egg and Spinach Sandwiches 42

18. Chicken, Potato, & Tarragon Bake 45

19. Tuna Stuffed Jacket Potatoes 48

20. Spicy Baked Chicken & Chips 50

21. Simple Cheesy Frittata 52

22. Risotto, Oven-Style 54

23. Chicken Stroganoff, Slow Cooker Style _____ *56*
24. Vegetable Mac 'n Cheese _____ *58*
25. Herby Tuna Balls with Spaghetti _____ *61*
26. Chicken Curry with Sweet Potato _____ *63*
27. Easy Chicken Kievs _____ *65*
28. Cheesy Tomato & Pasta Bake _____ *67*
29. Mushroom and Spinach Lasagna _____ *69*
30. Chickpea and Tomato Oven Bake _____ *71*
31. Cheesy Broccoli Soup _____ *73*
32. Super-Quick Black Beans and Rice _____ *75*
33. Lemon Zest Caper Pasta _____ *77*
34. Pork & Apple Burgers _____ *80*
35. Traditional Toad in The Hole _____ *82*
Conclusion _____ *84*
Final Words _____ *85*
Disclaimer _____ *87*

Introduction

Cooking for the whole family is a challenging task. Planning and keeping it healthy and delicious whilst being under a strict budget is difficult, especially if you have young kids at home.

When you are cooking in a daily basis, it is hard to actually have a variation with your cooking, and so, to prevent your family from getting bored with the same meals that you are cooking for them, you have to make sure you offer them different kinds of meals. Not so easy!

In these days and time, it is hard to cook up complicated meals all the time, so maybe save the prestige recipes for the weekends and cook up easy and affordable recipes during the weekdays. In that way you will be able to prevent your family from getting bored.

If you are worrying that you might not be able to find easy and affordable recipes, don't worry! In this book, allow me to show you quick, delicious and affordable meals that your family will surely enjoy. Learn from different techniques and explore different flavors from different parts of the world that will excite your palate. Add a few know-hows from simple tips given, and your cooking will be fun and enjoyable.

So, read on and step into the wonderful world of cooking. Make your life simple, and thrill your taste-buds at the same time! Happy cooking!

1. Green Beans in Coconut Milk

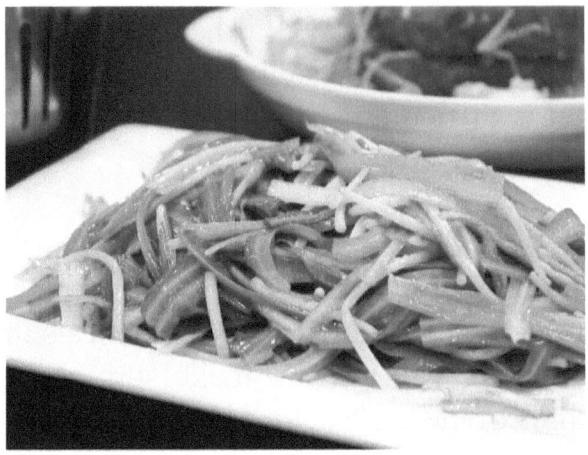

Green beans and the rich coconut milk flavor in this recipe complements well with the slight taste of chili. A good way of sharing this meal for the whole family as this not only whets the appetite but provides comforting taste and awakens the palate.

Ingredients

- 3 tablespoons of oil
- 2 cloves of garlic, chopped
- 1 small chopped onion
- 150 grams of ground pork
- 3 cups of green beans

- 1 can of coconut cream

- ½ cup of coconut milk

- 2 pieces of bird's eye chili, chopped

- Salt, pepper and sugar to taste

Method

1. Heat the oil in the pan. Sauté garlic and onions. Add the ground pork and cook thoroughly until brown.

2. Add the green beans and coconut cream. Simmer until liquid is reduced. Add coconut milk and cook until the beans are done and tender. Add chili. Season to taste. Serve hot and enjoy!

Tips

If you don't have any available fresh coconut cream and milk, powdered substitute will do for this recipe. The trick: dissolve them with the right amount of water and voila…you already have your coconut milk for this recipe.

2. Minestrone Soup with Macaroni

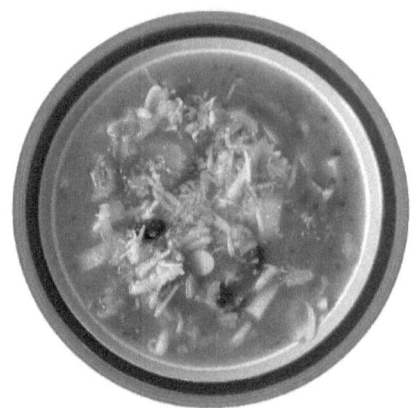

This is a complete meal in itself. It is definitely satisfying, comforting and tasty – most of all affordable and easy to prepare.

Ingredients

- 2 tablespoons of oil

- 4 cloves of minced garlic

- 1 onion (finely chopped)

- 1 red bell pepper (diced)

- 1 green bell pepper (diced)

- 1 zucchini (diced)

- ½ cup of mushroom (sliced)
- 4 cups of beef stock
- 1 cup of uncooked macaroni
- 1 can of white beans (drained)
- 1 pack of frozen mixed vegetables (small size)
- Fresh basil for garnish (chopped)

Method

1. Heat oil in a pot then sauté onions and garlic. Add red and green bell peppers, mushrooms and zucchini. Add the beef stock and bring it to a boil. Reduce heat.

2. Add macaroni pasta and cook until done. Add beans and the frozen vegetables then simmer for a few more minutes. Ladle into bowl then serve hot with chopped fresh basil on top. Enjoy!

Tips

Plain pasta, tortellini or shell pasta can also be a good substitute for this recipe.

3. Chili Beans with Pasta

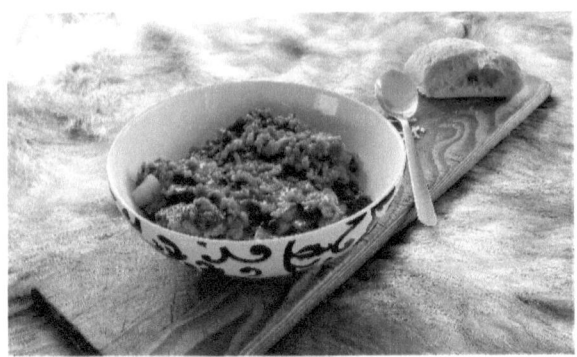

This is an easy recipe that you can prepare in just 20 minutes – a quick but delicious and nutritious meal for the whole family.

Ingredients

- 1 pound of ground beef (choose those that are lean)
- ¾ cup of onion (chopped)
- 1 15 oz. red kidney beans (drained and rinsed)
- 1 can of 14 ½ oz. diced tomatoes
- 1 can of 8 oz. tomato sauce
- ½ cup elbow macaroni (uncooked)
- 1 can of 4 oz. diced green chile peppers (drained)

- 2 teaspoons of chili powder

- ½ teaspoon of garlic salt

- ½ cup of shredded Monterey Jack (or you can use cheddar cheese)

Method

1. Cook the meat with the onions in a large skillet until brown and tender. Drain excess fat. Add the beans, diced tomatoes, macaroni, tomato sauce, chili powder, garlic salt and chile peppers. Bring to boil and then reduce heat.

2. Cover and simmer for about 20 minutes or until your macaroni if cooked. Stir often. Take out the skillet from the heat and sprinkle it with cheese. Cover and let stand for about 2 minutes. Serve and enjoy!

Tips

You can keep it kid-friendly by decreasing the amount of chili or whatever is preferred by your kids.

4. Tuna Spaghetti with Tomatoes and Garlic

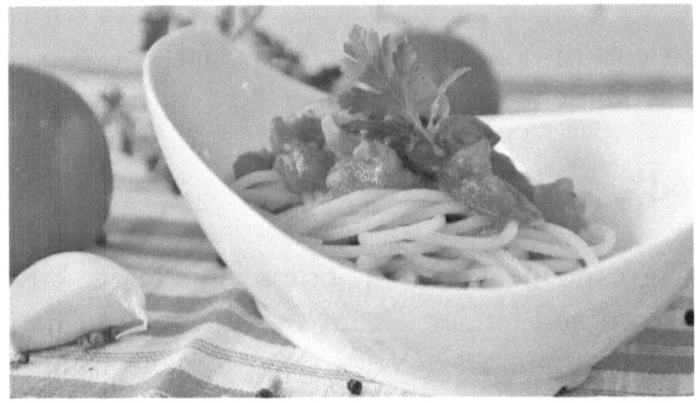

Here's another quick recipe that uses ingredients that are readily available in your pantry. Saves precious time but produces a delightful meal.

Ingredients

- 1 400-gram pack of spaghetti

- ¼ cup of olive oil

- 4 heads of garlic (chopped)

- 3-4 pieces of large, plump tomatoes (seeded and cut to strips)

- 2 cups of tuna (drained)

- Salt and pepper to taste

Method

1. Cook pasta according to label instructions. Drain and set aside. Heat your oil in the pan and sauté your garlic until it releases its aroma. Add the tomatoes and cook thoroughly.

2. Add the tuna and continue cooking until done. Add in the cooked pasta and toss them together. Add salt and pepper to taste. Serve and enjoy.

Tips

If you want to add a bit of spice in this dish, you can use the spicy kind of tuna. Tuna is rich in Omega 3 which is good for your heart.

5. Beef and Vegetable Stew

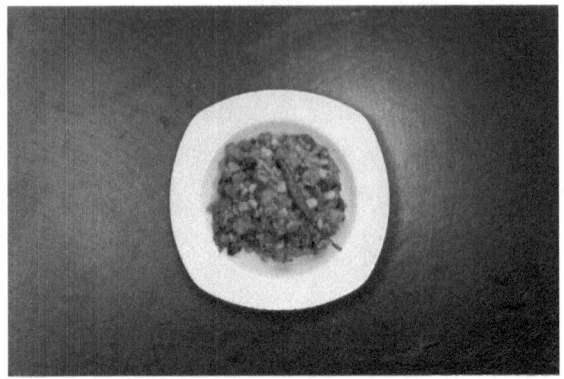

Try this protein rich and nutritious recipe that is hassle-free and budget friendly.

Ingredients

- 1 tablespoon of oil
- 2 tablespoons of garlic (chopped)
- 1 small onion (chopped)
- 500 grams of beef (cut into small cubes)
- 1 can of whole kernel corns (drained)
- 1 can of crushed tomatoes
- Salt and pepper to taste

- Spring onions (sliced to strips)

Method

1. Heat oil in a pan. Sauté onions and garlic. Add the beef and cook for a few minutes. Add the tomatoes and corn and simmer until the beef is already tender.

2. Reduce the sauce. Season with salt and pepper then add some sliced spring onions for garnish. Serve hot and enjoy.

Tips

You can use tender cut beef so that it would cook faster. Cut them into small and uniform size so that they will be cooked evenly and all at the same time. For some touch of herbs, you can replace the plain canned tomatoes with those that are already flavored. They are usually mixed with oregano and basil.

Read This FIRST - 100% FREE BONUS

FOR A LIMITED TIME ONLY – Get Olivia's best-selling book *"The #1 Cookbook: Over 170+ of the Most Popular Recipes Across 7 Different Cuisines!"* absolutely FREE!

Readers have absolutely loved this book because of the wide variety of recipes. It is highly recommended you check these recipes out and see what you can add to your home menu!

Once again, as a big thank-you for downloading this book, I'd like to offer it to you *100% FREE for a LIMITED TIME ONLY!*

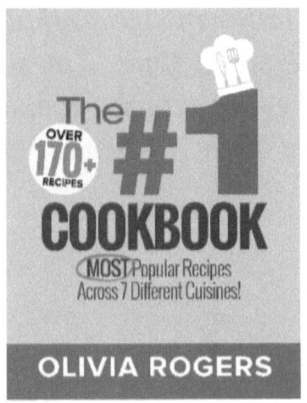

Get your free copy at:

TheMenuAtHome.com/Bonus

6. Garlic-Herb Beef Roast

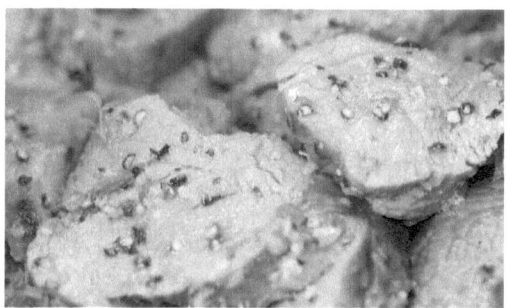

Another recipe that can be prepared in less than 30 minutes, easy to make and simple. It's a good source of protein and the addition of vegetables will provide the nutrients that your family needs.

Ingredients

- 1 oz. of beef roast au jus (refrigerated)
- 1 lb. of small red potatoes (quartered)
- 3 medium sized carrots (peeled and sliced diagonally)
- 1 tablespoon of cooking oil
- 3 tablespoons of fresh flatleaf parsley (chopped)
- 3 cloves of garlic (minced)
- 1 tablespoon of lemon peel (finely shredded)

Method

1. Cook and cover the beef roast in a large skillet over medium-high heat for about 10 minutes. Once done, simmer for another 5 minutes until its juices are reduced slightly.

2. Place the quartered potatoes and sliced carrots in a microwave safe dish. Drizzle the vegetables with oil and season with pepper. Toss slightly to even out the flavor and oil. Cover and cook inside the microwave oven on high temperature for about 10 minutes until its tender.

3. For the garlic-herb mixture, combine garlic, parsley and lemon peel in a bowl. Set aside. Stir the vegetables into the skillet with the beef roast. Place them on the serving plate and add some garlic-herb mixture. Serve hot and enjoy.

Tips

You can buy your beef roast au jus on any leading supermarkets. Add flair to this prepared meal by using this recipe instead of eating it as it is.

7. Paella in a Flash

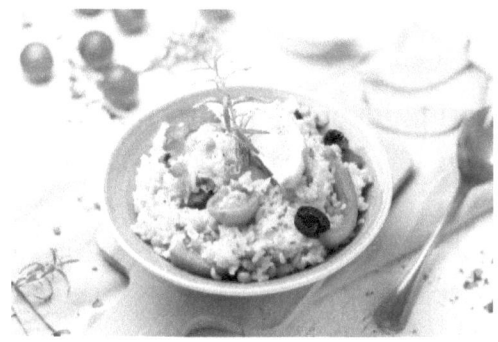

Paella is a rice dish that originated from Spain and became popular around the world. In this recipe, you will be able to prepare this dish in under 30 minutes. This preparation is already a complete and healthy meal in itself. Ingredients are easy to find and easy to use.

Ingredients

- ¼ cup of corn oil
- 1 teaspoon of annatto powder
- 1 tablespoon of garlic (minced)
- 1 cup of onions (chopped)
- 1 small red bell pepper (sliced)
- 3 pieces of Chorizo (sliced)

- 1 cup of chicken breast (cooked and sliced into cubes)
- ¼ teaspoon of Spanish paprika
- 2 pieces of chicken bouillon cube
- 3 ½ cups of cooked rice
- Salt and pepper to taste

Method

1. In a large sauce pan, heat oil and garlic and annatto powder. Mix the onions and bell peppers. Cook until fragrant. Add in the chorizo, paprika, chicken, and the bouillon cubes.

2. Cook until the cubes are already dissolved and incorporated in the dish. Add the cooked rice and mix well. Make sure that the color will be distributed evenly on the rice. Season with salt and pepper. Serve and enjoy.

Tips

For a richer and delightful tasting paella, you can add shrimps, mussels or squid. This would also add a festive flair in your paella.

8. Baked Mushroom-Chicken Curry Rice

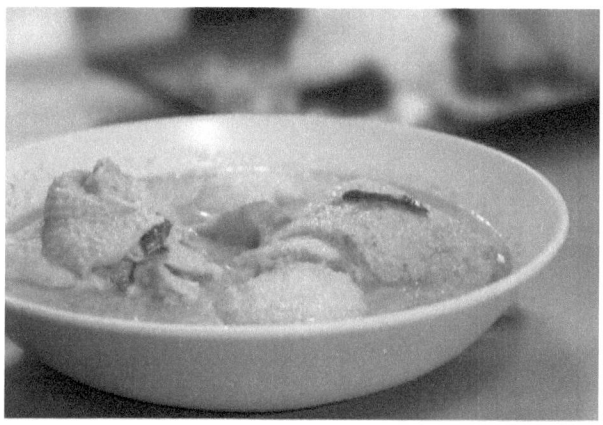

Under a tight budget? Then whip up this complete meal with your leftover ingredients and create a new and exciting dish any time.

Ingredients

- 1 can of condensed cream of mushroom soup
- ¼ cup of coconut milk
- 1/3 cup of water
- 3 tablespoons of butter
- 2 tablespoons of oil
- 3 cloves of garlic (chopped)

- 1 small onion (chopped)
- 1 chicken breast fillet (cubed)
- 6 pieces of button mushrooms (sliced)
- 2 teaspoons of curry powder
- 1 large tomato (cut to chunks)
- Salt and pepper to taste
- Mozzarella cheese (grated)

Method

1. Combine coconut milk, cream of mushroom and water in a bowl. Whisk until smooth and set aside. Heat the oil and butter together in a pan. Sauté the garlic and onions. Make sure that onions are already translucent. Cook chicken for about a minute then add the mushrooms, tomato chunks and curry powder. Mix well.

2. Add rice and combine them well to coat it evenly with the curry. Stir in the cream of mushroom mixture and mix well. Cook rice until it has a rich, creamy consistency. Add salt and pepper to taste.

3. Transfer to an ovenproof container and top it with the mozzarella cheese. Bake in a microwave oven for 2-

3 minutes on medium-high heat or until cheese melts. You can also bake it on a preheated oven with 350 degrees for about 10 minutes or until cheese melts. Serve hot and enjoy!

Tips

To save more time, you can replace your button mushrooms with canned mushrooms that are already sliced – it's fast and convenient.

9. Red Rice Soup with Beef

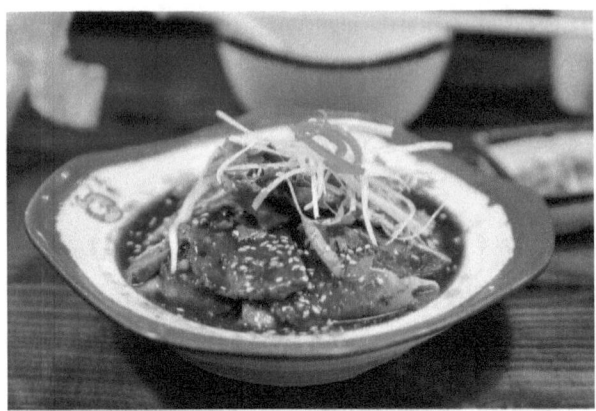

This is a simple yet nutritious comfort food that is definitely filling and heart-warming. You can make a large batch of this recipe and freeze in the refrigerator. Simply reheat once needed and you will have an instant comfort food meal available.

Ingredients

- 1 tablespoon of canola oil
- 2.2 lbs. of beef short ribs
- 1 large white onion (chopped)
- 6 cloves of garlic (crushed and chopped)
- ½ cup of carrots (chopped)

- ½ cup of celery (chopped)

- 12 cups of water

- 1 cup of red rice (uncooked)

- Salt and pepper for tasting

Method

1. Heat oil in a very large thick-bottomed pot until hot. Sear short ribs in batches and set aside on plate.

2. Using the same pot, sauté until translucent. Add garlic, celery, carrots and cook for a minute. Add the short ribs back in the pot and add in the water. Simmer until the ribs become soft and tender. Remove the ribs. Strain the stock and remove excess fat on top of the pot.

3. Transfer stock in another clean pot and bring to boil. Add the red rice and the ribs. Simmer and cook around 30 minutes or until rice is thoroughly cooked. Add salt and pepper to taste. Serve and enjoy.

Tips

If you want to shorten the cook time of your ribs, you can use a pressure cooker.

10. Stir-Fried Shrimp Hofan

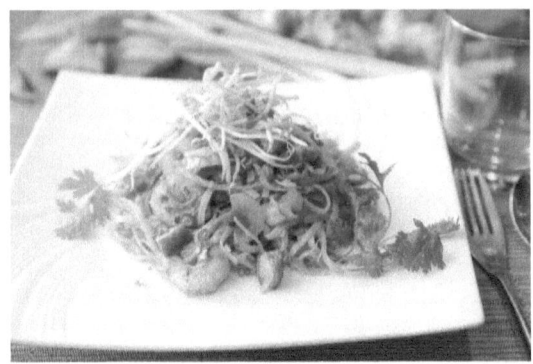

Asian cuisine is now becoming a popular choice among food lovers and consumers. In this recipe, learn to cook Asian and discover the style and its taste. This is another way of introducing healthy, simple and a new food idea to your family.

Ingredients

- 1 pack of Hofan noodles
- 4 tablespoons of oil
- 250 grams of shrimps (shelled and deveined)
- 1 cup of bean sprouts
- 1 cake of Tofu (deep fried and sliced into thick strips)
- 1-3 tablespoons of oyster sauce

- 2 eggs (beaten)

- 2 teaspoons of water

- Salt and pepper for tasting

- ½ cups of chives (cut into thin strips)

Method

1. Cook hofan noodles as per package instructions. Drain and add 2 tablespoons of oil to avoid noodles from sticking to one another. Pour remaining oil in a pan and sauté shrimps and bean sprouts. Add in the fried tofu. Pour the beaten eggs and let it set before mixing.

2. Mix in the oyster sauce with water and pour on the pan. Add salt and pepper to taste then add the chives. Put the noodles on a serving plate and top it with the shrimp-veggie mixture. Serve hot and enjoy!

Tips

Hofan or ho fen are flat Chinese noodles. They are the same with the Italian fettuccine and also to the vermicelli noodles which are found in most Pad Thai recipes.

11. Corned Beef Hearty Soup

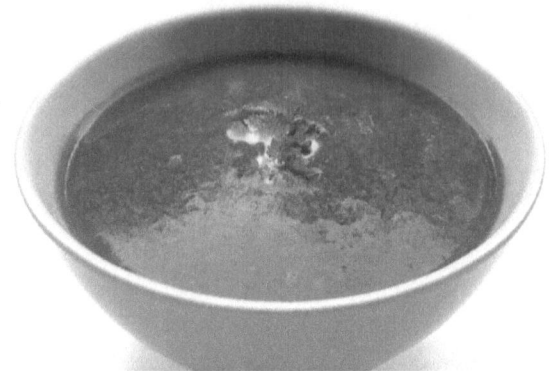

Hearty soups with soft and freshly-baked bread are perfect on any occasion. May it be for dinner or during cold seasons this recipe is proven to be filling but light on the budget.

Ingredients

- 1 tablespoon of oil

- 2 tablespoons of onions (sliced)

- 1 small can of chunky corned beef (any brand of your choice)

- 1 can of condensed cream of mushroom soup

- 1 cup of water

- 1 can of cream of corn

Method

1. Heat oil in a pot and sauté onion until translucent. Add the corned beef and cook until they are brown and a bit crusty.

2. Add in the cream of mushroom soup, cream of corn and water. Mix thoroughly and simmer around 5 minutes. Serve hot and provide bread.

Tips

Crusty artisan breads like sourdough, multigrain loaf or ciabatta are a perfect dipping combination with this deliciously thick soup.

12. Meatloaf Pasta Parmigiana

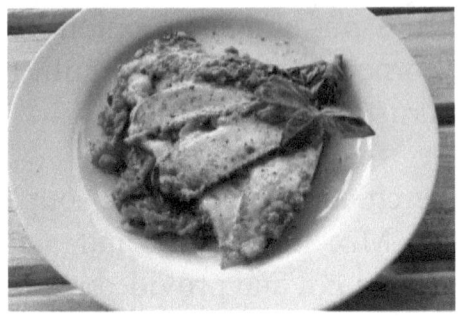

Here's a great way to use leftover meatloaf and turn it into an exciting dish for the whole family.

Ingredients

For the leftover meatloaf

- 1 cup of all-purpose flour
- 1 egg (beaten)
- 1 cup of breadcrumbs
- Oil to be used for frying
- ¼ cup of mozzarella cheese (grated)
- 1/3 cup of Parmesan cheese (grated)
- Cooked pasta

For the sauce

- 1 tablespoon of oil
- 1 tablespoon of garlic (minced)
- 1 small onion (diced)
- 1 big can of crushed tomatoes
- 1 teaspoon of dried oregano
- 1 teaspoon of dried basil
- ½ teaspoon of sugar
- Salt and pepper to taste

Method

1. Slice the leftover meatloaf then coat with flour. Dip them in beaten eggs followed by coating them on breadcrumbs. Set aside and chill for a short time. Heat the oil and cook the meatloaf until golden brown on both sides. Pat excess oil using paper towels. Set aside.

2. Heat oil then sauté onions and garlic in a saucepan. Add the tomatoes and simmer for about 10 minutes. Add more water if needed then mix in the herbs, salt and pepper.

3. Sprinkle top of fried meatloaf with the cheeses then broil them in an oven toaster or pre-heated oven. Check to see if the cheeses are already melted then remove and set aside.

4. Toss the cooked pasta with olive oil and season with garlic powder and salt. Plate the dish with cooked pasta then topped with the sauce and meatloaf Parmigiana. Serve immediately. You can add more cheese if you want. Enjoy!

Tips

You can also use the breaded leftover meatloaf to make a healthy sandwich for your kids to take to their school.

13. Luncheon Meat Katsudon

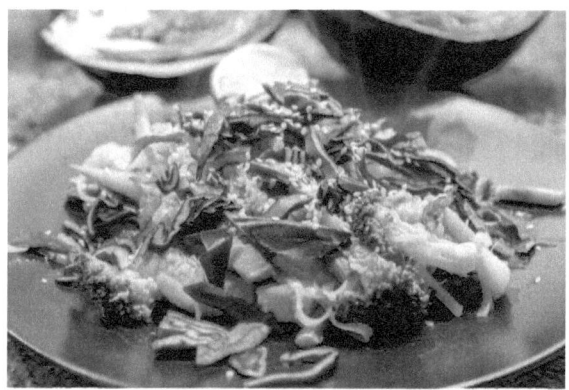

Here's another great way to use your leftover meatloaf. This time you can use another Asian flavor – let's travel in Japan. Elevate these simple canned goods into a great meal.

Ingredients

- 1 can of luncheon meat of your choice (cut them into ½ inch-thick slices)

- 1 cup all-purpose flour

- 2 eggs (beaten)

- 2 cups of Japanese bread crumbs

- Oil

- 4-6 cups of cooked rice

- 4-6 medium sized eggs
- Onion rings
- 1 medium sized carrots (julienned)
- Leeks or spring onion (chopped)

For the sauce

- 3 tablespoons of Kikkoman Soy Sauce
- ¼ cup of sugar
- beef bouillon cube, halved (optional)
- 2 cups of water

Method

1. Slice the leftover meatloaf then coat with flour. Dip them in beaten eggs followed by coating them on breadcrumbs. Heat the oil and cook the meatloaf until golden brown on both sides. Pat excess oil using paper towels. Set aside. Place all the ingredients for the sauce in a saucepan. Bring to boil and simmer for another 2 minutes.

2. Scoop a good amount of rice to individual bowls and top it with the fried meatloaf around 2- 3 slices will do. Make sure that the sauce is hot and ladle them to each of the

bowl. Break an egg on top of each bowl with the sauce and garnish with carrots, onion ring and spring onions. Serve and enjoy!

Tips

In making Katsudon, make sure that your sauce is piping hot to make sure that the eggs will be completely cooked on its own heat.

14. Seafood Fried Rice

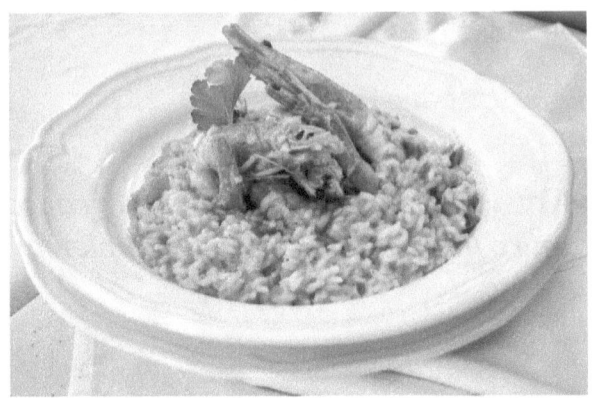

Try this complete meal in a flash. Increase your fiber and vitamin B intake with this delicious and convenient meal. Another Asian inspired meal that will surely satisfy your hungry family members.

Ingredients

- 2 tablespoons of canola oil (or peanut oil)

- 1 tablespoon of garlic (chopped)

- 2 tablespoons of onions (chopped)

- 2 tablespoons of spring onions (chopped)

- 1 Chinese sausage (cubed finely)

- 3 eggs (beaten)

- 12 cups of brown rice (cooked)
- ½ cup of shrimps
- ½ cup of clam meat
- ¼ cup of dried squid flakes (shredded)
- 3 tablespoons of soy sauce
- 1 teaspoon of sweet-chili sauce

Method

1. Heat oil in a large wok and sauté onions, garlic and spring onions until you can smell the fragrance. Combine the sausage with the beaten egg. Mix well until the eggs are thoroughly cooked

2. Add the other ingredients and stir-fry until shrimps change color and get cooked. Make sure that all of the ingredients are evenly combined with the rice. Serve hot and enjoy!

Tips

The secret to making an awesome fried rice is to make sure that all ingredients are mixed and combined well. So better get ready to stir, stir, stir!

15. Cajun Pork Chops with Gravy

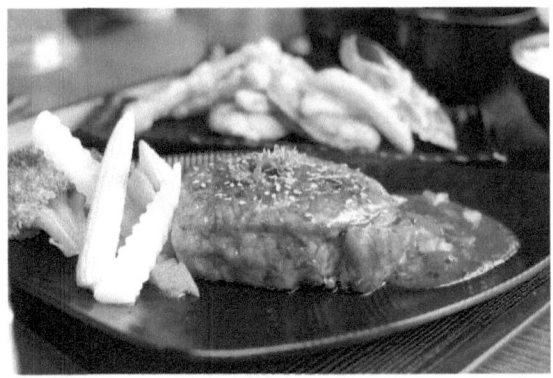

This is a proven family favorite in every home. Who can resist the tasty Cajun flavors topped with gravy? Come on and give it a try!

Ingredients

- 6 pieces of pork chops (choose the lean ones)
- 1 cup of onion (chopped)
- 1 cup of green pepper (chopped)
- 1 cup of celery (chopped)
- 1 cloves of garlic (crushed)
- 1 pack of beef gravy (prepared per package instructions)

- 3 cups of rice (cooked)
- Vegetable oil
- Cajun seasoning
- Salt and pepper to taste

Method

1. Rub the chops with Cajun seasonings liberally. Place a small amount of oil in the pan. Sear the chops and both sides then set aside. Put the onion, celery, garlic and pepper to the pan and sauté until fragrant.

2. Add the pork chops back into the pan and pour in the prepared gravy on it. Simmer for about 45 minutes. Serve hot over cooked rice and enjoy!

Tips

Cajun seasoning mostly consists of a blend of salt and variety of spices such as cayenne pepper and garlic.

16. Chicken Barbecue with Java Rice

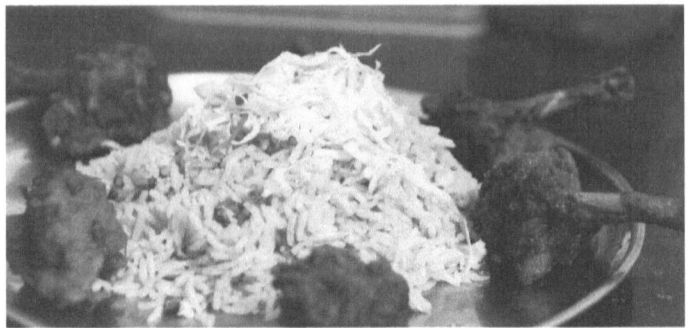

Tried and tested recipe that would bring satisfaction to your whole family. Every bite has a taste of sweet, tangy and juicy fillets combined with the perfect blend of java rice.

Ingredients

- 4 pieces of chicken breast fillet
- ½ cup of store bought barbecue marinade

For the java rice

- 3 tablespoons of annatto oil
- 1 teaspoon of garlic (minced)
- ¾ cup ground pork
- 4 cups of rice (cooked)

- Salt and pepper to taste

- Peanut sauce for dipping (optional)

Method

1. Combine chicken and barbecue marinade in a bowl for 2-4 hours. Place them on the refrigerator. Heat grill or you may use a grill pan, until it is very hot. Put the marinated chicken on the pan and cook for about 2-3 minutes on both sides. Make sure to lower the heat to avoid burning the chicken. Set aside.

2. In making the java rice: In the pan, heat the annatto oil. Sauté garlic and add the ground until cooked. Add the cooked rice and mix them well. Add salt and pepper to taste. Remove from the heat and set aside. Transfer the rice to a serving plate then place the barbecued chicken with the peanut sauce. Serve hot and enjoy!

Tips

Try marinating your chicken meat for 24 hours. This would allow more time for the marinade mix to be fully incorporated in the meat making it much tastier.

17. Egg and Spinach Sandwiches

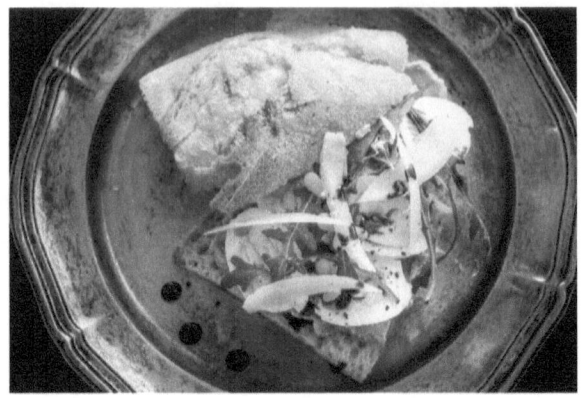

Thought that eggs are only good for breakfast? Guess again. Try out this recipe and it will surely make you want for more. Fast, delicious and healthy. It might make your kids eat vegetables too.

Ingredients

- 4 pieces of tomatoes (halved lengthwise)

- 4 pieces of English muffins (split)

- 2 ½ tablespoons of extra virgin olive oil

- ¼ red onion (thinly sliced)

- ¼ lbs. Canadian Bacon sliced (cut into thin strips)

- 8 cups of baby spinach

- 4 large eggs

- 1/3 cup of cheddar cheese

- Salt and pepper to taste

Method

1. Preheat your broiler. Arrange the tomatoes with the cut side up on a baking tray. Season them with salt and pepper. Broil them until they are soft for about 2 minutes. Remove it from the broiler. Place the English muffins on the baking tray and brush it with a tablespoon of olive oil then set aside.

2. Heat another tablespoon of olive oil in a nonstick pan over medium-high heat. Cook the onion until translucent around 2 minutes. Cook then the sliced Canadian bacon until slightly browned and add in the spinach until it turns wilted. Add salt and pepper to taste then transfer to them in a bowl and keep them warm.

3. Add the remaining ½ tablespoon of olive oil on the pan and cook the eggs sunny side up in the pan. Add salt and pepper to taste. Place the cheese on top of the tomatoes. Return them with the English muffin on the broiler and let the cheese melt. Separate the muffins on each plate and top it with the tomato, spinach and bacon mixture and add the fried egg. Place on top with broiled tomatoes. Serve and enjoy!

Tips

You can replace spinach with either kale, chard or collard greens. These veggies are also packed with the nutrients your body needs.

18. Chicken, Potato, & Tarragon Bake

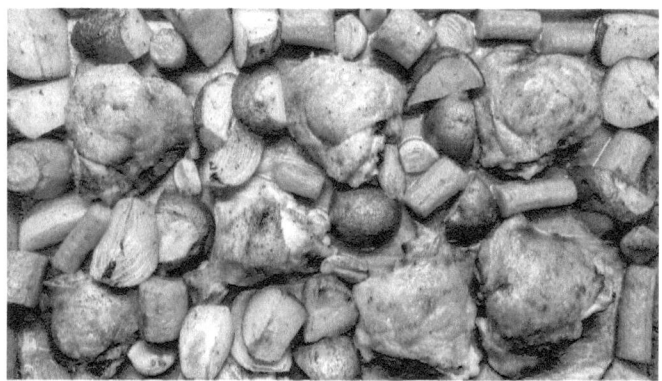

Potato is the staple of many family meal, and chicken is certainly a budget meat that everyone loves. Throw in some delicious and fragrant tarragon into this hearty and warming meal, for a sure-fire positive reaction!

Ingredients

- 60g unsalted butter
- 6 chicken thighs, boneless and cut into chunks
- 80g pancetta, smoked works best for flavor
- 2 onions, cut into slices
- 40g plain flour
- 500ml chicken stock

- 3 tablespoons of tarragon, chopped finely
- 3 tablespoons of wholegrain mustard
- 4 tablespoons of double cream
- 2 medium sized packs of pre-mashed potato (or make your own)
- A little olive oil

Method

1. Over a medium heat, melt 20g of the butter. Add the chicken and pancetta (cut into pieces) and fry for around 5 minutes, ensuring the chicken is cooked. Set the contents to one side, but keep the pan.

2. Add the rest of the butter to the pan and cook the onions until soft. Add the flour and stir well, leaving to cook for a couple of minutes. Remove the pan from the heat and add the chicken stock, mixing slowly.

3. Put the pan back on the heat and leave for 5 minutes. Add the tarragon, the cream, and the mustard and combine. Add the chicken and pancetta and leave to cook for a further 5 minutes. Preheat your grill to a high heat and warm up the mashed potato.

4. Take a casserole dish and layer your chicken mixture into the bottom. Over the top, add the potato and

ensure it reaches the edges. Drizzle a small amount of olive oil over the top. Place the dish under the grill for around 10 minutes.

Tips

If you're not a fan of pre-prepared mashed potato, you can go ahead and make your own just as easily, and probably cheaply!

19. Tuna Stuffed Jacket Potatoes

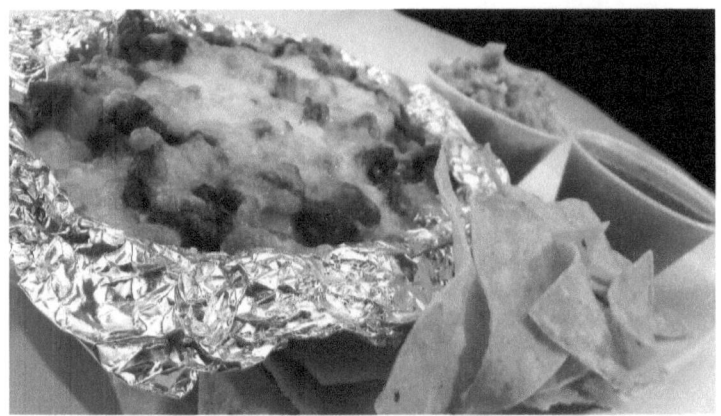

Jacket potatoes are not only a budget choice for families, but a real favorite too! This recipe has a slight twist on the theme, with healthier sweet potatoes taking the centre stage.

Ingredients

- 4 sweet potatoes

- 185g can of tuna, drained

- Half a red onion, sliced

- 1 small red chilli, sliced and deseeded

- The juice of 1 lime

- 6 tablespoons of Greek yoghurt

Method

1. Prepare the potatoes, cleaning them and pricking them thoroughly with a fork on all sides. Microwave the potatoes for around 20 minutes, until cooked.

2. Cut the potatoes in half and leave to cool a little. Separate the tuna a little in a dish and then divide over the top of each of the potato halves.

3. Divide the red onion between the potatoes, and do the same with the chilli. Squeeze a little lime juice over each half. Add a little Greek yogurt over each half.

Tips

Again, if you don't like sweet potato, you can opt for regular ones, and if you prefer a crispy skin to your jackets, pop them in the oven for the last ten minutes or so, to crisp them up nicely!

20. Spicy Baked Chicken & Chips

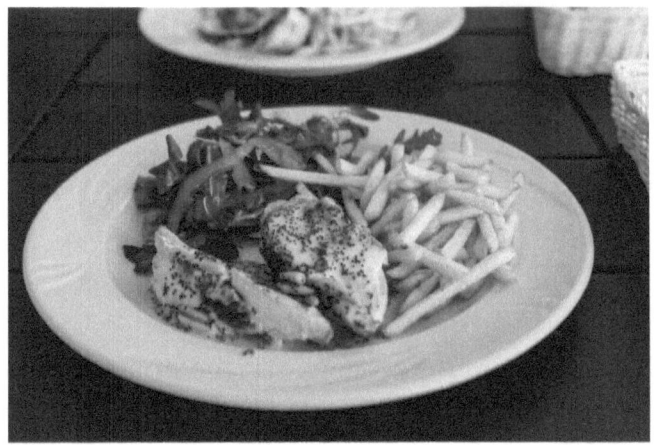

A modern twist on the old chicken and chips dish that your kids are sure to love! If you want to up the ante on the vegetable intake in your child's diet, throw some carrot and aubergine slices into the baking tray, to roast and serve alongside.

Ingredients

- 1 tablespoon of Cajun seasoning
- 2 tablespoons of oil, vegetable will be fine
- The zest and juice of 1 lime
- 750g potato, sliced into chips, as thick as you like
- 1kg of chicken wings

Method

1. Preheat your oven to 200 degrees. In a small mixing bowl, mix together the Cajun, the oil, the zest, and the juice. Toss the potato chips in the bowl and coat well.

2. Take a large baking tray and cover with foil to prepare. Place the chips on the tray, focusing around the outside.

3. Place the chicken in the middle of the tray. Bake in the oven for around 20 minutes. Turn the chips over and return back to the oven for another 20 minutes. Ensure the chicken is cooked before serving.

Tips

You can serve with your favorite dips or ketchup to add an extra dimension to the dish, and to make it extra healthy, serve with a green salad.

21. Simple Cheesy Frittata

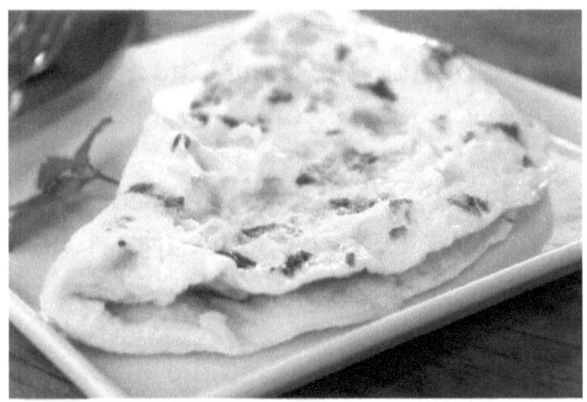

There is nothing simpler and more filling than a frittata, ideal for an impressive mid-week meal. Get the kids to help you too, as the recipe is easy enough for young chefs!

Ingredients

- 2 spring onions, chopped
- 4 tablespoons of peas, make sure they are defrosted well
- 1 courgette, grated
- 2 slices of lean ham
- 100g feta cheese
- 4 medium eggs

Method

1. Preheat the oven to 180 degrees. Combine the peas and chopped spring onion in a bowl. Add the grated courgette and combine it all together. Rip the ham into slices and combine everything together. Crumble the feta cheese into the bowl and combine.

2. In a separate bowl, crack the eggs and whisk them up. Pour the eggs into the bowl and mix together well.

3. Take an ovenproof dish and brush with oil to prevent sticking. Pour the mixture into the dish and place in the oven, cook for around half an hour, making sure the egg is set but not burnt.

Tips

If you want to bulk up this meal a little more, place some sliced potatoes in the oven alongside, or simply serve with a hearty green salad!

22. Risotto, Oven-Style

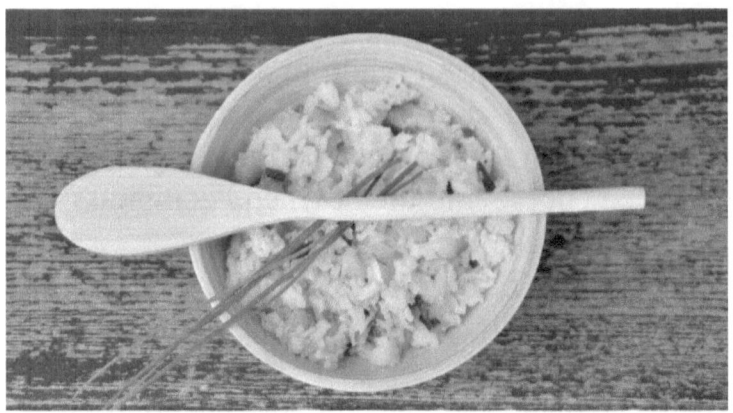

Your usual risotto is cooked in a pan over the hob, and it can be quite hard to get the right consistency; not this dish! Twist the usual risotto recipe a little and create a much easier style, and for a budget price too – most ingredients will already be in your store cupboard.

Ingredients

- 250g bacon, cut into small pieces

- 1 onion, chopped into small pieces

- 25g butter

- 300g risotto rice

- 150g cherry tomatoes, cut into halves

- 700ml chicken stock

- 50g grated Parmesan cheese

Method

1. Preheat the oven to 200 degrees. Over a medium heat, fry the bacon until crispy, for around 5 minutes. Add the onion and the butter and continue to cook for another few minutes.

2. Add the rice and combine everything together, cooking for a further 2 minutes. Add the stock and the tomatoes and stir really well. Cover the pan and place in the oven for around 18 minutes. Before serving, stir in the parmesan until melted.

Tips

If there are no children at home that night, you can add a little white wine to the dish, to make it a tad bit more luxurious! Half a glass of white wine will do the trick.

23. Chicken Stroganoff, Slow Cooker Style

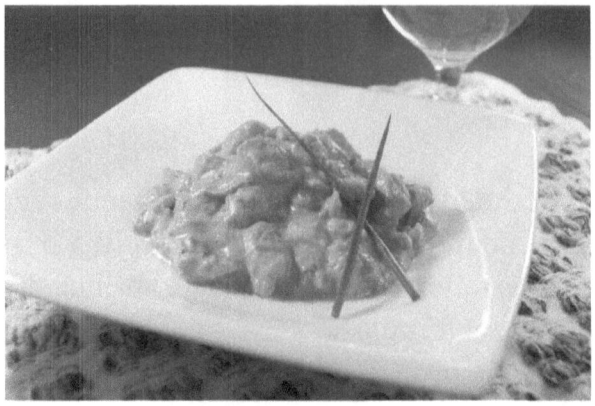

Slow cookers are a family cooking godsend, and you can easily add this to your cooker and leave it until you're ready to return home from work and feed the masses. Simple, hearty, and ideal for the colder months.

Ingredients

- 2 tablespoons of olive oil
- 1 chopped onion
- 4 chicken breasts, cut into cubes
- 300g mushrooms, cut into halves
- 1 can of condensed chicken soup
- 150ml of chicken stock

- 1 teaspoon of paprika

- 100ml of sour cream

- 15g chives, cut into small pieces

Method

1. Over a medium heat, warm up the oil in a large pan. Add the chicken breasts to the pan. Now, add the onions and cook for around 5 minutes, turning the chicken over at the halfway mark and stirring regularly.

2. Take your slow cooker and place the content of the frying pan inside. Add the mushrooms, the soup, the stock, sour cream, and the paprika.

3. Combine the ingredients together well. Put the lid on the slow cooker and set to low for 5-6 hours. Once cooked, sprinkle over the chives and serve.

Tips

Add a little tagliatelle pasta to the dish for an extra treat. Simply cook just before you are ready to serve the chicken stroganoff.

24. Vegetable Mac 'n Cheese

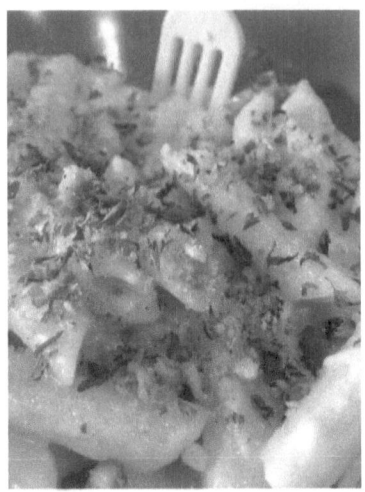

We all know how hard it can be to pack vegetables into the diets of your family members, and this traditional, well-loved, classic meal is a fantastic way to smuggle in a few fresh veggies!

Ingredients

- 150g cubed butternut squash
- 300g penne pasta
- 40g butter
- 1 leek, cut into slices
- 25g flour

- 600ml milk

- 100g peas, defrosted

- 175g Cheddar cheese

- Breadcrumbs made from 1 slice of brown bread

Method

1. Preheat the oven to 200 degrees. Steam the butternut squash in boiling water for around 20 minutes, until it is totally tender. Once cooked, drain and put into a food processor and blitz to form a smooth consistency. Meanwhile, cook the pasta to your liking.

2. In a medium pan, and over a medium heat, melt the butter. Add the leek and cook for 2 minutes. Add the flour and combine, cooking for a further 2 minutes. Remove the pan from the heat and whisk the milk inside, gradually.

3. Put the pan back onto the heat and bring to the boil, stirring constantly. Allow the mixture to simmer for 5 minutes. Add the peas, stir, and simmer again. Remove the pan from the heat and add the butternut squash. Add the majority of the cheese and stir in well. Add the pasta and combine well.

4. Take a large ovenproof dish and transfer the mixture into it. Sprinkle the rest of the cheese over the top of the dish and then add the breadcrumbs, distributing evenly. Bake in the oven for 20 minutes, until golden brown and bubbly.

Tips

Serve with crusty, warm bread for a truly luxurious, midweek feast.

25. Herby Tuna Balls with Spaghetti

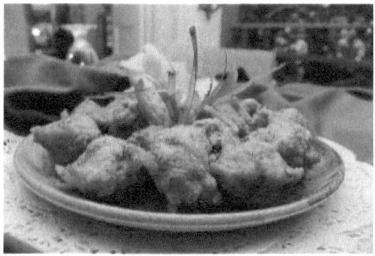

Do you love fish cakes? This twist on the old recipe is Italian-style, and also much cheaper, thanks to using a can of tuna that you're sure to have in your cupboard already!

Ingredients

- 2 regular cans of tuna, 160g if possible

- A few pine nuts

- The zest of 1 lemon

- A few parsley leaves, chopped

- 50g breadcrumbs

- 1 egg, beaten

- 400g spaghetti

- A jar of pasta sauce, 500g if possible

Method

1. Drain the tuna and flake into a bowl- keeping the oil from the tuna to one side. Add the pine nuts, zest, parsley, beaten egg, and the breadcrumbs and combine.

2. Time to get your hands dirty! Use your hands to form balls of the mixture, around the size of a walnut, you should get 12 from the mixture. Meanwhile, cook the spaghetti to your liking.

3. Over a medium heat, warm up the oil from the tuna in a frying pan. Fry the balls for 5 minutes, turning over halfway, and checking they don't burn. Place on kitchen roll and blot to remove the excess oil.

4. In another saucepan, warm up the tomato sauce. Once cooked, toss the tuna balls, the pasta, and the tomato sauce together and serve.

Tips

If you want to bulk up the meal, or add in a few extra vitamins, add peppers and onions to the tomato sauce – a sneaky way to hide some veggies!

26. Chicken Curry with Sweet Potato

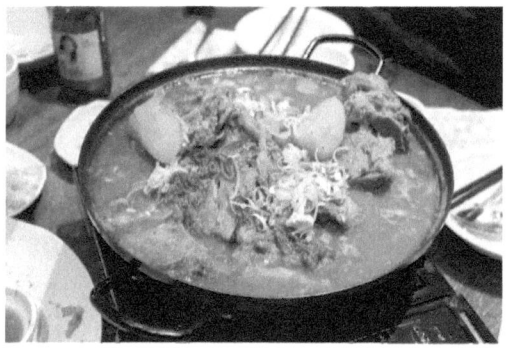

A traditional favorite – most people love a good chicken curry! To add extra nutrition to this delicious dish, sweet potato is added, whilst being super quick and easy too!

Ingredients

- 1 tablespoon of sunflower oil
- 1 onion, chopped into small pieces
- 450g chicken thighs, cut into chunks
- 165g jar of Korma paste
- 2 crushed garlic cloves
- 500g sweet potato, cut into cubes
- 400g can of tomatoes, chopped ones work best

- 100g spinach

- Basmati rice

Method

1. In a medium pan, heat the oil. Cook the onion over a low heat until soft for around 5 minutes. Turn up the heat a little and add into the pan the chicken, cooking until browned. Add the korma paste and garlic, and cook for a further 2 minutes.

2. Now add 100ml of water and combine well. Add the potatoes and the tomatoes, and combine again. Simmer for around half an hour, ensuring that the chicken is cooked properly, and that the potato is soft.

3. Add the spinach to the pan and combine. Remove the pan from the heat and continue to stir the contents until the spinach is totally wilted. Meanwhile, cook the rice according to packet instructions. Serve together!

Tips

Warm up some packet naan breads if you want to create a real Indian restaurant vibe! This meal is ideal for a Saturday night alternative to an expensive takeaway.

27. Easy Chicken Kievs

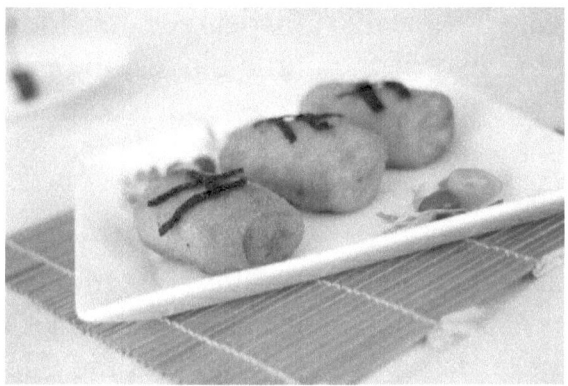

Chicken kievs are renowned for being difficult, but not this recipe! Try this delicious, herby dish for a mid-week treat, served with potato or green salad. Something a little different!

Ingredients

- 6 peeled garlic cloves
- A few leaves of parsley
- 85g breadcrumbs
- 4 chicken breasts, boneless and skinless
- 4 tablespoons of soft cheese with garlic
- 4 tablespoons of olive oil

Method

1. Preheat your oven to 200 degrees. In a food processer, combine two of the garlic cloves, the parsley, and a tablespoon of the olive oil. Once combined, add the breadcrumbs and season with salt and pepper. Pulse until well combined.

2. Tip the breadcrumb mix onto a medium sized plate. Take each chicken breast and cut a 2-inch slit into one side of each – it is best to do it at the thicker end, to prevent splitting.

3. Into each slit, add a quarter of the soft cheese, and press together the edges, to stop the cheese from oozing out. Rub a little oil over the chicken and dab them onto the plate with the herby mixture, on both sides to coat.

4. Take a roasting tray and arrange the chicken inside. Place the rest of the garlic cloves inside and drizzle over the remaining oil. Put into the oven and bake for around 25 minutes. Serve whilst still warm.

Tips

Before serving, squeeze the kiev a little to allow the garlic butter to pool on the plate – delicious!

28. Cheesy Tomato & Pasta Bake

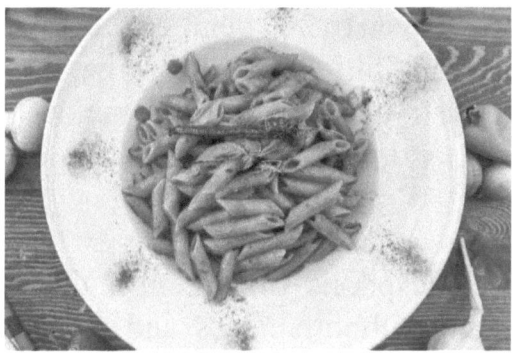

If you're running towards month end and cash is a little low, this hearty, tasty, and downright delicious dish is the perfect dinner answer!

Ingredients

- 400g pasta of your choice
- 190g jar of pesto with sundried tomatoes
- 2 chillies, chopped and deseeded
- 1 large chopped tomato
- 1 teaspoon of paprika, smoked if possible
- 50g Parmesan cheese, grated
- 150g goat's cheese, chopped into small pieces

Method

1. Preheat the oven to 200 degrees. Meanwhile, cook the pasta to your liking. Take a large, ovenproof dish. Into the dish, add the chillis, tomatoes, paprika, and the pesto, and combine well – keep the pesto jar to one side.

2. Add 3 tablespoons of water to the empty jar, to remove any stubborn pieces, and add to the ovenproof dish. Combine everything well. Once the pasta is cooked and drained, add that to the dish also. Add half of the Parmesan cheese and mix everything together.

3. Distribute the goat's cheese evenly over the dish, and the rest of the parmesan. Cook in the oven for around 20 minutes, until the cheese is bubbling.

Tips

If you don't want the dish super-spicy, you can use just one chilli or omit them entirely.

29. Mushroom and Spinach Lasagna

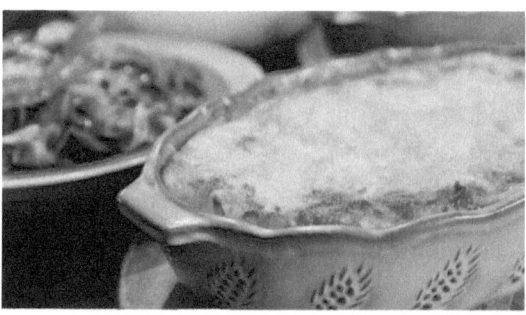

Another fantastic dish that everyone loves, but with a truly different twist! Omit the meat and go with spinach and mushrooms instead for a healthy way to enjoy this classic Italian dish.

Ingredients

- 1 tablespoon olive oil
- 1 crushed garlic clove
- 250g mushrooms, cut into thin slices
- 1 teaspoon of chopped thyme leaves
- A medium bag of spinach, usually around 200g
- 300g soft cheese
- 4 tablespoons of Parmesan cheese, grated

- 6 lasagna sheets

Method

1. Preheat the oven to 200 degrees. In a large pan, heat up the oil and cook the garlic for 1 minute. Add the thyme and mushrooms, cooking for around 3 minutes. Add the spinach, and stir until wilted.

2. Remove the pan from the heat and add the soft cheese, stirring to combine. Add 1 tablespoon of the Parmesan cheese and combine. Take a medium baking dish and spread a quarter of the spinach/cheese mixture in the bottom.

3. Add two lasagna sheets on top and then add more mixture, and more lasagna sheets, until everything has been used up. The rest of the Parmesan can be sprinkled over the top. Bake in the oven for 35 minutes.

Tips

If you want to really up the Italian vibe for your evening meal, serve with a oven baked garlic baguette, as a treat on the side!

30. Chickpea and Tomato Oven Bake

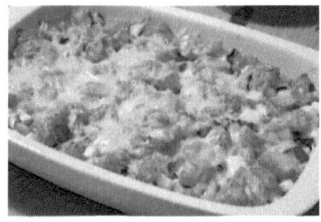

Healthy, delicious, cheap, and super-easy – what could be better than this quick and hearty dish? If you want to omit the bread it healthier, you can, but the bread adds a true crispy dimension!

Ingredients

- 1 cubed aubergine
- 1 chopped onion
- 2 tablespoons of olive oil
- 1 chopped garlic clove
- 400g chopped tomatoes
- 2 teaspoons of oregano, dried
- 200g halved cherry tomatoes
- 1 medium can of drained chickpeas

- 4 baguette slices

- 3 tablespoons of grated Parmesan cheese

Method

1. Preheat the oven to 200 degrees. In a large frying pan, over a medium heat, fry the onion and the aubergine for around 5 minutes. Next, add the chopped tomatoes and the garlic and combine.

2. Add 1 cup of water and combine. Add half of the oregano and combine. Bring the mixture to the boil, turn it down and allow it to simmer for around 10 minutes.

3. Add the cherry tomatoes and the chickpeas for the last 2 minutes, and combine well. Take a large baking dish and pour the mixture inside. Take the bread and brush both sides with a little of the oil.

4. Take the rest of the oregano and Parmesan cheese and combine together, pouring over the bread. Place the bread over the oven dish mixture and place in the oven for around 20 minutes.

Tips

Garnish with a little basil if you want a true Italian taste to this dish.

31. Cheesy Broccoli Soup

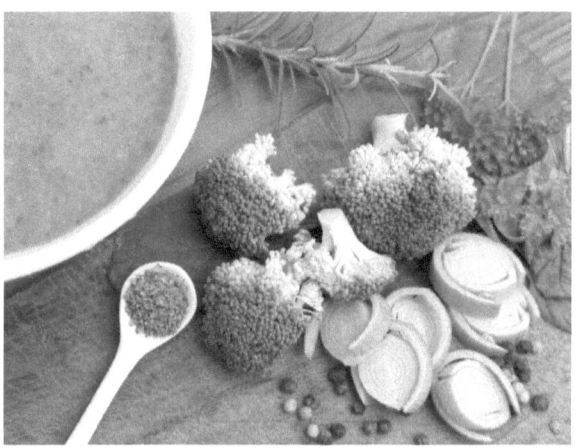

Cold winter evenings are designed for homemade soup and crusty bread, whilst the leftovers can be warmed up the next day for lunch – twice the cost effectiveness, and super-healthy too!

Ingredients

- 2 broccoli heads, chopped

- 1 small piece of Parmesan cheese, cut into smaller chunks

- A little grated Parmesan for serving

- 1 tablespoon of soy sauce

- 1 tablespoon of lemon juice

Method

1. In a medium sized saucepan, bring 2 cups of water to the boil. Add the broccoli and the pieces of Parmesan and stir until the cheese melts. Add the soy sauce. Cover the pan and allow to simmer for around 8 minutes, ensuring the broccoli is tender.

2. Use a handheld blender to combine the ingredients. Add the lemon juice and stir. Season with salt and pepper. Serve with the grated Parmesan over the top of the dish.

Tips

If you want an extra cheesy taste to your soup, use Parmesan with rind on the side, as this will give you extra flavor overall.

32. Super-Quick Black Beans and Rice

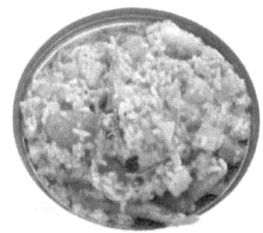

This is another dish which can be made and reheated for lunch the next day. This dish can easily last for two days, allowing you to send the kids to school with something a little different in their pack up!

Ingredients

- 2 teaspoons of canola oil

- 1 chopped onion

- 1 chopped garlic clove

- 1 teaspoon of ground cumin

- 1 teaspoon of ground chilli powder

- 2oz can of roasted chilli peppers, green are best

- 2 cups of rice, cooked

- ¼ cup of red sofrito – easily found in the Latin section of most supermarkets

- 1 can of black beans, drained

- ¼ teaspoon of Kosher salt

- ¼ teaspoon of black pepper

Method

1. Over a medium heat, take a large frying pan and cook the onion until soft. Add the garlic, cumin, chilli powder, green peppers, and cook for around 2 minutes.

2. Add the rice to the pan and combine well, cooking for around 3 minutes, until the rice is warm. Add the sofrito and black beans and combine well. Add a little salt and pepper and combine again. Serve warm or refrigerate.

Tips

If you want to store the dish for later consumption, you can keep it for two days. Simply add a tiny bit of water to break it up, and warm up in the microwave for a couple of minutes.

33. Lemon Zest Caper Pasta

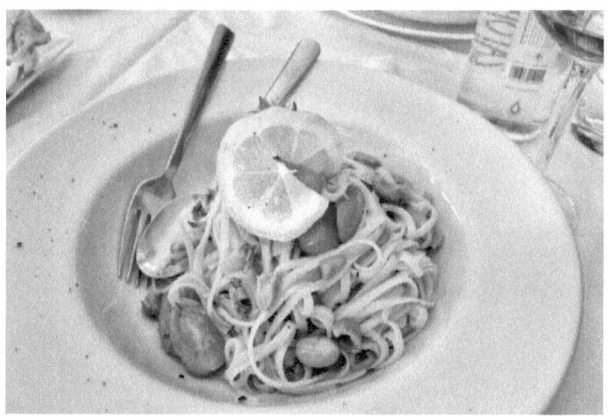

Pasta doesn't have to involve tomato sauces and beef, and this lemony twist to pasta with capers is a totally different dish to try, and one which is sure to be a hit with the family.

Ingredients

- 1lb of pasta shells

- 1 tablespoon of olive oil

- 1 cup of fresh breadcrumbs

- The zest of 1 lemon

- 2 tablespoons of chopped parsley

- 2 tablespoons of grated Parmesan

- Kosher salt

- Ground black pepper

- 3 tablespoons of butter

- 4 minced garlic cloves

- ¼ cup of capers

- The juice of 1 lemon

Method

1. Boil the pasta to your liking. Meanwhile, toast the breadcrumbs until crispy.

2. In a large frying pan, over a medium heat, warm up the oil and sauté the lemon zest and breadcrumbs, for around 4 minutes. Remove from the head and add the parsley, salt, a little pepper, and the parmesan combining together well, placing in another bowl.

3. In the same pan, melt the butter and add the garlic, cooking for around a minute. Remove from the heat again and add the capers and lemon juice, combining well. Keep a quarter of the pasta water, but drain the rest.

4. Put the frying pan back on a medium heat and add the pasta water, pasta, and the lemon caper mixture,

cooking for a couple of minutes, until the pasta water has disappeared. Add a quarter of the breadcrumb mixture and toss. Serve with the rest of the breadcrumbs as a garnish.

Tips

You can easily store anything leftover in the refrigerator for 5 days, provided it is kept in a container which is airtight.

34. Pork & Apple Burgers

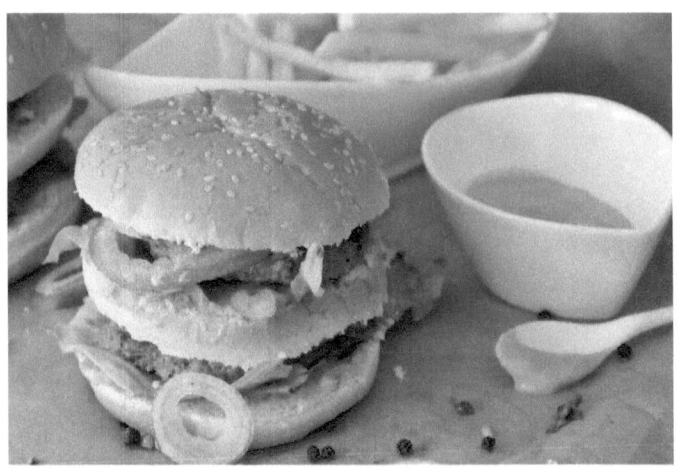

A different twist on the usual beef burger, and something the kids will love! Again, a boost of vitamins from the apples, and they won't even notice! To add to the health side of it, there is no excessive frying in sight.

Ingredients

- 750g of pork mince
- 75g of breadcrumbs
- 2 teaspoons of finely chopped sage
- 1 grated apple, dessert apples work much better
- 2 chopped spring onions

- 1 beaten egg

- Salt

- Ground black pepper

Method

1. Preheat the oven to 190 degrees. Take a baking tray and cover it with foil. Take a large mixing bowl and combine the pork, salt, and pepper. Using your hands, combine together into a large bowl, and separate in half.

2. Place one half into a bowl and cover it over, leaving it in the refrigerator until you are going to cook it – you can leave it for 2 days maximum. The rest of the mixture should be divided into four equal sized burgers, using your hands.

3. Heat up the oil in a frying pan and cook quickly on each side for one minute, until brown. Remove from the heat and place the burgers onto the baking tray. Cook in the oven for 15 minutes.

Tips

Serve with burger buns, mustard, thick cut tomato, red onion, and pickle for a true burger experience!

35. Traditional Toad in The Hole

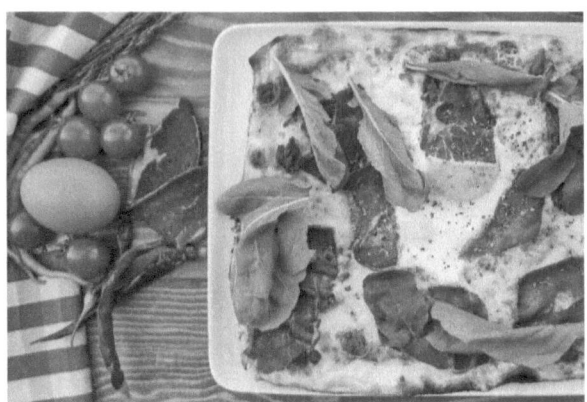

Everyone has heard of it, not everyone knows how to make it, but it is the ideal budget meal for a family. All you need is gravy, instant if you want, and there you have it – the ideal meal for everyone to enjoy.

Ingredients

- 8 pork sausages

- 1 tablespoon of vegetable oil

- 225g of plain flour

- 4 medium eggs

- 250ml milk

- Salt

- Pepper

Method

1. Preheat the oven to 200 degrees. Take a large baking dish and add the oil to the bottom, to prevent burning. Now, take the sausages and arrange them in the bottom of the dish, in one layer. Place the dish in the oven for 10 minutes.

2. In a medium bowl combine together the eggs, flour, and half of the milk, to form a smooth consistency. Slowly mix in the rest of the milk to create a batter. Season the batter with salt and pepper.

3. Take the baking dish out of the oven and pour the batter mixture over the top, covering the dish by three quarters. Place the dish back in the oven and cook for 35 minutes. The dish is cooked when it is brown and has risen.

Tips

Make this dish healthier by serving with a few vegetables!

Conclusion

This book of 35 quick, easy, and truly delicious recipes is designed to help you serve fantastic recipes every single night of the week, whist keeping your outgoings to a minimum. In addition, none of these recipes are laden with fat or particular unhealthy, so they are ideal for a busy family, or for those who are trying to watch their waist line a little!

None of these ingredients are particularly exotic or out of the ordinary, and can all be found easily in your local supermarket, or within your store cupboard already. Every one of these recipes will serve a family of four on average, and you can add basics as a side, such as salad or potatoes, if you want to increase your portion size.

All that's really left to decide is which one you're going to try first!

Final Words

I would like to thank you for downloading my book and I hope I have been able to help you and educate you about something new.

If you have enjoyed this book and would like to share your positive thoughts, could you please take 30 seconds of your time to go back and give me a review on my Amazon book page!

I greatly appreciate seeing these reviews because it helps me share my hard work!

Again, thank you and I wish you all the best with your cooking journey!

Last Chance to Get YOUR Bonus!

FOR A LIMITED TIME ONLY – Get Olivia's best-selling book *"The #1 Cookbook: Over 170+ of the Most Popular Recipes Across 7 Different Cuisines!"* absolutely FREE!

Readers have absolutely loved this book because of the wide variety of recipes. It is highly recommended you check these recipes out and see what you can add to your home menu!

Once again, as a big thank-you for downloading this book, I'd like to offer it to you *100% FREE for a LIMITED TIME ONLY!*

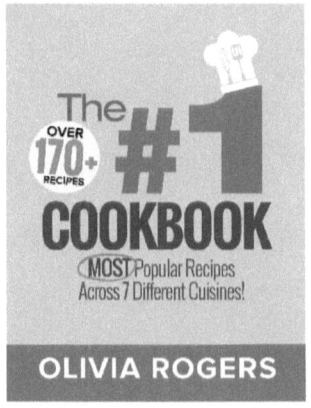

Get your free copy at:

TheMenuAtHome.com/Bonus

Disclaimer

This book and related site provides recipe and food advice in an informative and educational manner only, with information that is general in nature and that is not specific to you, the reader. The contents of this book and related site are intended to assist you and other readers in your personal efforts. Consult your physician or nutritionist regarding the applicability of any information provided in our information to you.

Nothing in this book should be construed as personal advice or diagnosis, and must not be used in this manner. The information provided about conditions is general in nature. This information does not cover all possible uses, actions, precautions, side-effects, or interactions of medicines, or medical procedures. The information in this site should not be considered as complete and does not cover all diseases, ailments, physical conditions, or their treatment.

No Warranties: The authors and publishers don't guarantee or warrant the quality, accuracy, completeness, timeliness, appropriateness or suitability of the information in this book, or of any product or services referenced by this site.

The information in this site is provided on an "as is" basis and the authors and publishers make no representations or warranties of any kind with respect to this information. This site may contain inaccuracies, typographical errors, or other errors.

Liability Disclaimer: The publishers, authors, and other parties involved in the creation, production, provision of information, or delivery of this site specifically disclaim any responsibility, and shall not be held liable for any damages, claims, injuries, losses, liabilities, costs, or obligations including any direct, indirect, special, incidental, or consequences damages (collectively known as "Damages") whatsoever and howsoever caused, arising out of, or in connection with the use or misuse of the site and the information contained within it, whether such Damages arise in contract, tort, negligence, equity, statute law, or by way of other legal theory.

www.ingramcontent.com/pod-product-compliance
Lightning Source LLC
Chambersburg PA
CBHW021129080526
44587CB00012B/1203